Sugar? Nah, I Am Sweet Enough

Date: 12/7/19

Weight: ______

Daily Goal: ______

	Calories	Carbs (g)	Sugars (g)	Fiber (g)	Protien (g)	Fat (g)
Breakfast: Real #123 @ 7:10 Am (Asm #88) Time: ______						
Lunch: Time: ______						
Dinner: Time: ______						
Page Totals:						

Sleep: ____________________

Water: ____________________

Mood: ____________________

	Calories	Carbs (g)	Sugars (g)	Fiber (g)	Protien (g)	Fat (g)
Other Meals / Snacks:						
Page Totals:						

Blood Sugar Log	Before	After	Insulin	Meds
Breakfast				
Lunch				
Dinner				

Activity • Exercise	Duration	Calories	Intensity

Other Notes, Vitamins, Supplements Meds:

____

____

____

____

Date: ____________

Weight: ____________

Daily Goal: ____________

	Calories	Carbs (g)	Sugars (g)	Fiber (g)	Protien (g)	Fat (g)
Breakfast: Time: ______						
Lunch: Time: ______						
Dinner: Time: ______						
Page Totals:						

Sleep: ____________________

Water: ____________________

Mood: ____________________

	Calories	Carbs (g)	Sugars (g)	Fiber (g)	Protien (g)	Fat (g)
Other Meals / Snacks:						
Page Totals:						

Blood Sugar Log	Before	After	Insulin	Meds
Breakfast				
Lunch				
Dinner				

Activity • Exercise	Duration	Calories	Intensity

Other Notes, Vitamins, Supplements Meds:

____

____

____

____

Date: ______________

Weight: ______________

Daily Goal: ______________

	Calories	Carbs (g)	Sugars (g)	Fiber (g)	Protien (g)	Fat (g)
Breakfast: Time: ______						
Lunch: Time: ______						
Dinner: Time: ______						
Page Totals:						

Sleep: ____________________

Water: ____________________

Mood: ____________________

	Calories	Carbs (g)	Sugars (g)	Fiber (g)	Protien (g)	Fat (g)
Other Meals / Snacks:						
Page Totals:						

Blood Sugar Log	Before	After	Insulin	Meds
Breakfast				
Lunch				
Dinner				

Activity • Exercise	Duration	Calories	Intensity

Other Notes, Vitamins, Supplements Meds:

____

____

____

____

Date: ______________

Weight: ______________

Daily Goal: ______________

	Calories	Carbs (g)	Sugars (g)	Fiber (g)	Protien (g)	Fat (g)
Breakfast: Time: ________						
Lunch: Time: ________						
Dinner: Time: ________						
Page Totals:						

Sleep: ______________________

Water: ______________________

Mood: ______________________

Other Meals / Snacks:	Calories	Carbs (g)	Sugars (g)	Fiber (g)	Protien (g)	Fat (g)
Page Totals:						

Blood Sugar Log	Before	After	Insulin	Meds
Breakfast				
Lunch				
Dinner				

Activity • Exercise	Duration	Calories	Intensity

Other Notes, Vitamins, Supplements Meds:

____

____

____

____

Date: ____________

Weight: ____________

Daily Goal: ____________

	Calories	Carbs (g)	Sugars (g)	Fiber (g)	Protien (g)	Fat (g)
Breakfast: Time: ______						
Lunch: Time: ______						
Dinner: Time: ______						
Page Totals:						

Sleep: ____________________

Water: ____________________

Mood: ____________________

	Calories	Carbs (g)	Sugars (g)	Fiber (g)	Protien (g)	Fat (g)
Other Meals / Snacks:						
Page Totals:						

Blood Sugar Log	Before	After	Insulin	Meds
Breakfast				
Lunch				
Dinner				

Activity • Exercise	Duration	Calories	Intensity

Other Notes, Vitamins, Supplements Meds:

____

____

____

____

Date: ____________

Weight: ____________

Daily Goal: ____________

	Calories	Carbs (g)	Sugars (g)	Fiber (g)	Protien (g)	Fat (g)
Breakfast: Time: ______						
Lunch: Time: ______						
Dinner: Time: ______						
Page Totals:						

Sleep: ____________________

Water: ____________________

Mood: ____________________

	Calories	Carbs (g)	Sugars (g)	Fiber (g)	Protien (g)	Fat (g)
Other Meals / Snacks:						
Page Totals:						

Blood Sugar Log	Before	After	Insulin	Meds
Breakfast				
Lunch				
Dinner				

Activity • Exercise	Duration	Calories	Intensity

Other Notes, Vitamins, Supplements Meds:

____

____

____

____

Date: ____________

Weight: ____________

Daily Goal: ____________

	Calories	Carbs (g)	Sugars (g)	Fiber (g)	Protien (g)	Fat (g)
Breakfast: Time: ______						
Lunch: Time: ______						
Dinner: Time: ______						
Page Totals:						

Sleep: ______________________

Water: ______________________

Mood: ______________________

	Calories	Carbs (g)	Sugars (g)	Fiber (g)	Protien (g)	Fat (g)
Other Meals / Snacks:						
Page Totals:						

Blood Sugar Log	Before	After	Insulin	Meds
Breakfast				
Lunch				
Dinner				

Activity • Exercise	Duration	Calories	Intensity

Other Notes, Vitamins, Supplements Meds:

____

____

____

____

Date: ______________

Weight: ______________

Daily Goal: ______________

	Calories	Carbs (g)	Sugars (g)	Fiber (g)	Protien (g)	Fat (g)
Breakfast: Time: ________						
Lunch: Time: ________						
Dinner: Time: ________						
Page Totals:						

Sleep: ____________________

Water: ____________________

Mood: ____________________

	Calories	Carbs (g)	Sugars (g)	Fiber (g)	Protien (g)	Fat (g)
Other Meals / Snacks:						
Page Totals:						

Blood Sugar Log	Before	After	Insulin	Meds
Breakfast				
Lunch				
Dinner				

Activity • Exercise	Duration	Calories	Intensity

Other Notes, Vitamins, Supplements Meds:

____

____

____

____

Date: ______________

Weight: ______________

Daily Goal: ______________

	Calories	Carbs (g)	Sugars (g)	Fiber (g)	Protien (g)	Fat (g)
Breakfast: Time: ________						
Lunch: Time: ________						
Dinner: Time: ________						
Page Totals:						

Sleep: ______________________

Water: ______________________

Mood: ______________________

	Calories	Carbs (g)	Sugars (g)	Fiber (g)	Protien (g)	Fat (g)
Other Meals / Snacks:						
Page Totals:						

Blood Sugar Log	Before	After	Insulin	Meds
Breakfast				
Lunch				
Dinner				

Activity • Exercise	Duration	Calories	Intensity

Other Notes, Vitamins, Supplements Meds:

____

____

____

____

Date: ____________

Weight: ____________

Daily Goal: ____________

	Calories	Carbs (g)	Sugars (g)	Fiber (g)	Protien (g)	Fat (g)
Breakfast: Time: ______						
Lunch: Time: ______						
Dinner: Time: ______						
Page Totals:						

Sleep: ______________________

Water: ______________________

Mood: ______________________

	Calories	Carbs (g)	Sugars (g)	Fiber (g)	Protien (g)	Fat (g)
Other Meals / Snacks:						
Page Totals:						

Blood Sugar Log	Before	After	Insulin	Meds
Breakfast				
Lunch				
Dinner				

Activity • Exercise	Duration	Calories	Intensity

Other Notes, Vitamins, Supplements Meds:

____

____

____

____

Date: ____________________

Weight: ____________________

Daily Goal: ____________________

	Calories	Carbs (g)	Sugars (g)	Fiber (g)	Protien (g)	Fat (g)
Breakfast: Time: ________						
Lunch: Time: ________						
Dinner: Time: ________						
Page Totals:						

Sleep: ____________________

Water: ____________________

Mood: ____________________

	Calories	Carbs (g)	Sugars (g)	Fiber (g)	Protien (g)	Fat (g)
Other Meals / Snacks:						
Page Totals:						

Blood Sugar Log	Before	After	Insulin	Meds
Breakfast				
Lunch				
Dinner				

Activity • Exercise	Duration	Calories	Intensity

Other Notes, Vitamins, Supplements Meds:

____

____

____

____

Date: ______________

Weight: ______________

Daily Goal: ______________

	Calories	Carbs (g)	Sugars (g)	Fiber (g)	Protien (g)	Fat (g)
Breakfast: Time: ________						
Lunch: Time: ________						
Dinner: Time: ________						
Page Totals:						

Sleep: ____________________

Water: ____________________

Mood: ____________________

	Calories	Carbs (g)	Sugars (g)	Fiber (g)	Protien (g)	Fat (g)
Other Meals / Snacks:						
Page Totals:						

Blood Sugar Log	Before	After	Insulin	Meds
Breakfast				
Lunch				
Dinner				

Activity • Exercise	Duration	Calories	Intensity

Other Notes, Vitamins, Supplements Meds:

____

____

____

____

Date: ____________

Weight: ____________

Daily Goal: ____________

	Calories	Carbs (g)	Sugars (g)	Fiber (g)	Protien (g)	Fat (g)
Breakfast: Time: ______						
Lunch: Time: ______						
Dinner: Time: ______						
Page Totals:						

Sleep: ____________________

Water: ____________________

Mood: ____________________

	Calories	Carbs (g)	Sugars (g)	Fiber (g)	Protien (g)	Fat (g)
Other Meals / Snacks:						
Page Totals:						

Blood Sugar Log	Before	After	Insulin	Meds
Breakfast				
Lunch				
Dinner				

Activity • Exercise	Duration	Calories	Intensity

Other Notes, Vitamins, Supplements Meds:

____

____

____

____

Date: ____________

Weight: ____________

Daily Goal: ____________

	Calories	Carbs (g)	Sugars (g)	Fiber (g)	Protien (g)	Fat (g)
Breakfast: Time: ______						
Lunch: Time: ______						
Dinner: Time: ______						
Page Totals:						

Sleep: ____________________

Water: ____________________

Mood: ____________________

	Calories	Carbs (g)	Sugars (g)	Fiber (g)	Protien (g)	Fat (g)
Other Meals / Snacks:						
Page Totals:						

Blood Sugar Log	Before	After	Insulin	Meds
Breakfast				
Lunch				
Dinner				

Activity • Exercise	Duration	Calories	Intensity

Other Notes, Vitamins, Supplements Meds:

____

____

____

____

Date: ______________

Weight: ______________

Daily Goal: ______________

	Calories	Carbs (g)	Sugars (g)	Fiber (g)	Protien (g)	Fat (g)
Breakfast: Time: ______						
Lunch: Time: ______						
Dinner: Time: ______						
Page Totals:						

Sleep: ______________________

Water: ______________________

Mood: ______________________

Other Meals / Snacks:	Calories	Carbs (g)	Sugars (g)	Fiber (g)	Protien (g)	Fat (g)
Page Totals:						

Blood Sugar Log	Before	After	Insulin	Meds
Breakfast				
Lunch				
Dinner				

Activity • Exercise	Duration	Calories	Intensity

Other Notes, Vitamins, Supplements Meds:

____

____

____

____

Date: ____________

Weight: ____________

Daily Goal: ____________

	Calories	Carbs (g)	Sugars (g)	Fiber (g)	Protien (g)	Fat (g)
Breakfast: Time: ______						
Lunch: Time: ______						
Dinner: Time: ______						
Page Totals:						

Sleep: ____________________

Water: ____________________

Mood: ____________________

	Calories	Carbs (g)	Sugars (g)	Fiber (g)	Protien (g)	Fat (g)
Other Meals / Snacks:						
Page Totals:						

Blood Sugar Log	Before	After	Insulin	Meds
Breakfast				
Lunch				
Dinner				

Activity • Exercise	Duration	Calories	Intensity

Other Notes, Vitamins, Supplements Meds:

____

____

____

____

Date: ______________

Weight: ______________

Daily Goal: ______________

	Calories	Carbs (g)	Sugars (g)	Fiber (g)	Protien (g)	Fat (g)
Breakfast: Time: ________						
Lunch: Time: ________						
Dinner: Time: ________						
Page Totals:						

Sleep: ____________________

Water: ____________________

Mood: ____________________

	Calories	Carbs (g)	Sugars (g)	Fiber (g)	Protien (g)	Fat (g)
Other Meals / Snacks:						
Page Totals:						

Blood Sugar Log	Before	After	Insulin	Meds
Breakfast				
Lunch				
Dinner				

Activity • Exercise	Duration	Calories	Intensity

Other Notes, Vitamins, Supplements Meds:

Date: ______________

Weight: ______________

Daily Goal: ______________

	Calories	Carbs (g)	Sugars (g)	Fiber (g)	Protien (g)	Fat (g)
Breakfast: Time: ________						
Lunch: Time: ________						
Dinner: Time: ________						
Page Totals:						

Sleep: ____________________

Water: ____________________

Mood: ____________________

	Calories	Carbs (g)	Sugars (g)	Fiber (g)	Protien (g)	Fat (g)
Other Meals / Snacks:						
Page Totals:						

Blood Sugar Log	Before	After	Insulin	Meds
Breakfast				
Lunch				
Dinner				

Activity • Exercise	Duration	Calories	Intensity

Other Notes, Vitamins, Supplements Meds:

____

____

____

____

Date: ________________

Weight: ________________

Daily Goal: ________________

	Calories	Carbs (g)	Sugars (g)	Fiber (g)	Protien (g)	Fat (g)
Breakfast: Time: ________						
Lunch: Time: ________						
Dinner: Time: ________						
Page Totals:						

Sleep: ______________________

Water: ______________________

Mood: ______________________

	Calories	Carbs (g)	Sugars (g)	Fiber (g)	Protien (g)	Fat (g)
Other Meals / Snacks:						
Page Totals:						

Blood Sugar Log	Before	After	Insulin	Meds
Breakfast				
Lunch				
Dinner				

Activity • Exercise	Duration	Calories	Intensity

Other Notes, Vitamins, Supplements Meds:

____

____

____

____

Date: ____________

Weight: ____________

Daily Goal: ____________

	Calories	Carbs (g)	Sugars (g)	Fiber (g)	Protien (g)	Fat (g)
Breakfast: Time: ________						
Lunch: Time: ________						
Dinner: Time: ________						
Page Totals:						

Sleep: ____________________

Water: ____________________

Mood: ____________________

Other Meals / Snacks:	Calories	Carbs (g)	Sugars (g)	Fiber (g)	Protien (g)	Fat (g)
Page Totals:						

Blood Sugar Log	Before	After	Insulin	Meds
Breakfast				
Lunch				
Dinner				

Activity • Exercise	Duration	Calories	Intensity

Other Notes, Vitamins, Supplements Meds:

____

____

____

____

Date: ______________

Weight: ______________

Daily Goal: ______________

	Calories	Carbs (g)	Sugars (g)	Fiber (g)	Protien (g)	Fat (g)
Breakfast: Time: ______						
Lunch: Time: ______						
Dinner: Time: ______						
Page Totals:						

Sleep: ____________________

Water: ____________________

Mood: ____________________

	Calories	Carbs (g)	Sugars (g)	Fiber (g)	Protien (g)	Fat (g)
Other Meals / Snacks:						
Page Totals:						

Blood Sugar Log	Before	After	Insulin	Meds
Breakfast				
Lunch				
Dinner				

Activity • Exercise	Duration	Calories	Intensity

Other Notes, Vitamins, Supplements Meds:

____

____

____

____

Date: ________________

Weight: ________________

Daily Goal: ________________

	Calories	Carbs (g)	Sugars (g)	Fiber (g)	Protien (g)	Fat (g)
Breakfast: Time: ________						
Lunch: Time: ________						
Dinner: Time: ________						
Page Totals:						

Sleep: ____________________

Water: ____________________

Mood: ____________________

	Calories	Carbs (g)	Sugars (g)	Fiber (g)	Protien (g)	Fat (g)
Other Meals / Snacks:						
Page Totals:						

Blood Sugar Log	Before	After	Insulin	Meds
Breakfast				
Lunch				
Dinner				

Activity • Exercise	Duration	Calories	Intensity

Other Notes, Vitamins, Supplements Meds:

____

____

____

____

Date: ____________

Weight: ____________

Daily Goal: ____________

	Calories	Carbs (g)	Sugars (g)	Fiber (g)	Protien (g)	Fat (g)
Breakfast: Time: ______						
Lunch: Time: ______						
Dinner: Time: ______						
Page Totals:						

Sleep: ______________________

Water: ______________________

Mood: ______________________

Other Meals / Snacks:	Calories	Carbs (g)	Sugars (g)	Fiber (g)	Protien (g)	Fat (g)
Page Totals:						

Blood Sugar Log	Before	After	Insulin	Meds
Breakfast				
Lunch				
Dinner				

Activity • Exercise	Duration	Calories	Intensity

Other Notes, Vitamins, Supplements Meds:

____

____

____

____

Date: ________________

Weight: ________________

Daily Goal: ________________

	Calories	Carbs (g)	Sugars (g)	Fiber (g)	Protien (g)	Fat (g)
Breakfast: Time: ________						
Lunch: Time: ________						
Dinner: Time: ________						
Page Totals:						

Sleep: ____________________

Water: ____________________

Mood: ____________________

	Calories	Carbs (g)	Sugars (g)	Fiber (g)	Protien (g)	Fat (g)
Other Meals / Snacks:						
Page Totals:						

Blood Sugar Log	Before	After	Insulin	Meds
Breakfast				
Lunch				
Dinner				

Activity • Exercise	Duration	Calories	Intensity

Other Notes, Vitamins, Supplements Meds:

____

____

____

____

Date: ______________

Weight: ______________

Daily Goal: ______________

	Calories	Carbs (g)	Sugars (g)	Fiber (g)	Protien (g)	Fat (g)
Breakfast: Time: ______						
Lunch: Time: ______						
Dinner: Time: ______						
Page Totals:						

Sleep: ____________________

Water: ____________________

Mood: ____________________

	Calories	Carbs (g)	Sugars (g)	Fiber (g)	Protien (g)	Fat (g)
Other Meals / Snacks:						
Page Totals:						

Blood Sugar Log	Before	After	Insulin	Meds
Breakfast				
Lunch				
Dinner				

Activity • Exercise	Duration	Calories	Intensity

Other Notes, Vitamins, Supplements Meds:

____

____

____

____

Date: ______________

Weight: ______________

Daily Goal: ______________

	Calories	Carbs (g)	Sugars (g)	Fiber (g)	Protien (g)	Fat (g)
Breakfast: Time: ______						
Lunch: Time: ______						
Dinner: Time: ______						
Page Totals:						

Sleep: ____________________

Water: ____________________

Mood: ____________________

	Calories	Carbs (g)	Sugars (g)	Fiber (g)	Protien (g)	Fat (g)
Other Meals / Snacks:						
Page Totals:						

Blood Sugar Log	Before	After	Insulin	Meds
Breakfast				
Lunch				
Dinner				

Activity • Exercise	Duration	Calories	Intensity

Other Notes, Vitamins, Supplements Meds:

____

____

____

____

Date: ______________

Weight: ______________

Daily Goal: ______________

	Calories	Carbs (g)	Sugars (g)	Fiber (g)	Protien (g)	Fat (g)
Breakfast: Time: ______						
Lunch: Time: ______						
Dinner: Time: ______						
Page Totals:						

Sleep: ____________________

Water: ____________________

Mood: ____________________

Other Meals / Snacks:	Calories	Carbs (g)	Sugars (g)	Fiber (g)	Protien (g)	Fat (g)
Page Totals:						

Blood Sugar Log	Before	After	Insulin	Meds
Breakfast				
Lunch				
Dinner				

Activity • Exercise	Duration	Calories	Intensity

Other Notes, Vitamins, Supplements Meds:

____

____

____

____

Date: ________________

Weight: ________________

Daily Goal: ________________

	Calories	Carbs (g)	Sugars (g)	Fiber (g)	Protien (g)	Fat (g)
Breakfast: Time: ________						
Lunch: Time: ________						
Dinner: Time: ________						
Page Totals:						

Sleep: ____________________

Water: ____________________

Mood: ____________________

Other Meals / Snacks:	Calories	Carbs (g)	Sugars (g)	Fiber (g)	Protien (g)	Fat (g)
Page Totals:						

Blood Sugar Log	Before	After	Insulin	Meds
Breakfast				
Lunch				
Dinner				

Activity • Exercise	Duration	Calories	Intensity

Other Notes, Vitamins, Supplements Meds:

____

____

____

____

Date: ____________

Weight: ____________

Daily Goal: ____________

	Calories	Carbs (g)	Sugars (g)	Fiber (g)	Protien (g)	Fat (g)
Breakfast: Time: ______						
Lunch: Time: ______						
Dinner: Time: ______						
Page Totals:						

Sleep: ______________________

Water: ______________________

Mood: ______________________

Other Meals / Snacks:	Calories	Carbs (g)	Sugars (g)	Fiber (g)	Protien (g)	Fat (g)
Page Totals:						

Blood Sugar Log	Before	After	Insulin	Meds
Breakfast				
Lunch				
Dinner				

Activity • Exercise	Duration	Calories	Intensity

Other Notes, Vitamins, Supplements Meds:

____

____

____

____

Date: ____________

Weight: ____________

Daily Goal: ____________

	Calories	Carbs (g)	Sugars (g)	Fiber (g)	Protien (g)	Fat (g)
Breakfast: Time: ______						
Lunch: Time: ______						
Dinner: Time: ______						
Page Totals:						

Sleep: ____________________

Water: ____________________

Mood: ____________________

	Calories	Carbs (g)	Sugars (g)	Fiber (g)	Protien (g)	Fat (g)
Other Meals / Snacks:						
Page Totals:						

Blood Sugar Log	Before	After	Insulin	Meds
Breakfast				
Lunch				
Dinner				

Activity • Exercise	Duration	Calories	Intensity

Other Notes, Vitamins, Supplements Meds:

____

____

____

____

Date: ______________

Weight: ______________

Daily Goal: ______________

	Calories	Carbs (g)	Sugars (g)	Fiber (g)	Protien (g)	Fat (g)
Breakfast: Time: ________						
Lunch: Time: ________						
Dinner: Time: ________						
Page Totals:						

Sleep: ____________________

Water: ____________________

Mood: ____________________

Other Meals / Snacks:	Calories	Carbs (g)	Sugars (g)	Fiber (g)	Protien (g)	Fat (g)
Page Totals:						

Blood Sugar Log	Before	After	Insulin	Meds
Breakfast				
Lunch				
Dinner				

Activity • Exercise	Duration	Calories	Intensity

Other Notes, Vitamins, Supplements Meds:

____

____

____

____

Date: ________________

Weight: ________________

Daily Goal: ________________

	Calories	Carbs (g)	Sugars (g)	Fiber (g)	Protien (g)	Fat (g)
Breakfast: Time: _______						
Lunch: Time: _______						
Dinner: Time: _______						
Page Totals:						

Sleep: ____________________

Water: ____________________

Mood: ____________________

	Calories	Carbs (g)	Sugars (g)	Fiber (g)	Protien (g)	Fat (g)
Other Meals / Snacks:						
Page Totals:						

Blood Sugar Log	Before	After	Insulin	Meds
Breakfast				
Lunch				
Dinner				

Activity • Exercise	Duration	Calories	Intensity

Other Notes, Vitamins, Supplements Meds:

____

____

____

____

Date: ______________

Weight: ______________

Daily Goal: ______________

	Calories	Carbs (g)	Sugars (g)	Fiber (g)	Protien (g)	Fat (g)
Breakfast: Time: ________						
Lunch: Time: ________						
Dinner: Time: ________						
Page Totals:						

Sleep: ____________________

Water: ____________________

Mood: ____________________

	Calories	Carbs (g)	Sugars (g)	Fiber (g)	Protien (g)	Fat (g)
Other Meals / Snacks:						
Page Totals:						

Blood Sugar Log	Before	After	Insulin	Meds
Breakfast				
Lunch				
Dinner				

Activity • Exercise	Duration	Calories	Intensity

Other Notes, Vitamins, Supplements Meds:

____

____

____

____

Date: ______________

Weight: ______________

Daily Goal: ______________

	Calories	Carbs (g)	Sugars (g)	Fiber (g)	Protien (g)	Fat (g)
Breakfast: Time: ______						
Lunch: Time: ______						
Dinner: Time: ______						
Page Totals:						

Sleep: ____________________

Water: ____________________

Mood: ____________________

	Calories	Carbs (g)	Sugars (g)	Fiber (g)	Protien (g)	Fat (g)
Other Meals / Snacks:						
Page Totals:						

Blood Sugar Log	Before	After	Insulin	Meds
Breakfast				
Lunch				
Dinner				

Activity • Exercise	Duration	Calories	Intensity

Other Notes, Vitamins, Supplements Meds:

____

____

____

____

Date: ____________

Weight: ____________

Daily Goal: ____________

	Calories	Carbs (g)	Sugars (g)	Fiber (g)	Protien (g)	Fat (g)
Breakfast: Time: ______						
Lunch: Time: ______						
Dinner: Time: ______						
Page Totals:						

Sleep: ______________________

Water: ______________________

Mood: ______________________

	Calories	Carbs (g)	Sugars (g)	Fiber (g)	Protien (g)	Fat (g)
Other Meals / Snacks:						
Page Totals:						

Blood Sugar Log	Before	After	Insulin	Meds
Breakfast				
Lunch				
Dinner				

Activity • Exercise	Duration	Calories	Intensity

Other Notes, Vitamins, Supplements Meds:

____

____

____

____

Date: ____________________

Weight: ____________________

Daily Goal: ____________________

	Calories	Carbs (g)	Sugars (g)	Fiber (g)	Protien (g)	Fat (g)
Breakfast: Time: ________						
Lunch: Time: ________						
Dinner: Time: ________						
Page Totals:						

Sleep: ____________________

Water: ____________________

Mood: ____________________

Other Meals / Snacks:	Calories	Carbs (g)	Sugars (g)	Fiber (g)	Protien (g)	Fat (g)
Page Totals:						

Blood Sugar Log	Before	After	Insulin	Meds
Breakfast				
Lunch				
Dinner				

Activity • Exercise	Duration	Calories	Intensity

Other Notes, Vitamins, Supplements Meds:

____

____

____

____

Date: ______________

Weight: ______________

Daily Goal: ______________

	Calories	Carbs (g)	Sugars (g)	Fiber (g)	Protien (g)	Fat (g)
Breakfast: Time: ______						
Lunch: Time: ______						
Dinner: Time: ______						
Page Totals:						

Sleep: ____________________

Water: ____________________

Mood: ____________________

Other Meals / Snacks:	Calories	Carbs (g)	Sugars (g)	Fiber (g)	Protien (g)	Fat (g)
Page Totals:						

Blood Sugar Log	Before	After	Insulin	Meds
Breakfast				
Lunch				
Dinner				

Activity • Exercise	Duration	Calories	Intensity

Other Notes, Vitamins, Supplements Meds:

Date: ____________

Weight: ____________

Daily Goal: ____________

	Calories	Carbs (g)	Sugars (g)	Fiber (g)	Protien (g)	Fat (g)
Breakfast: Time: ________						
Lunch: Time: ________						
Dinner: Time: ________						
Page Totals:						

Sleep: ____________________

Water: ____________________

Mood: ____________________

	Calories	Carbs (g)	Sugars (g)	Fiber (g)	Protien (g)	Fat (g)
Other Meals / Snacks:						
Page Totals:						

Blood Sugar Log	Before	After	Insulin	Meds
Breakfast				
Lunch				
Dinner				

Activity • Exercise	Duration	Calories	Intensity

Other Notes, Vitamins, Supplements Meds:

____

____

____

____

Date: ______________

Weight: ______________

Daily Goal: ______________

	Calories	Carbs (g)	Sugars (g)	Fiber (g)	Protien (g)	Fat (g)
Breakfast: Time: ______						
Lunch: Time: ______						
Dinner: Time: ______						
Page Totals:						

Sleep: ____________________

Water: ____________________

Mood: ____________________

Other Meals / Snacks:	Calories	Carbs (g)	Sugars (g)	Fiber (g)	Protien (g)	Fat (g)
Page Totals:						

Blood Sugar Log	Before	After	Insulin	Meds
Breakfast				
Lunch				
Dinner				

Activity • Exercise	Duration	Calories	Intensity

Other Notes, Vitamins, Supplements Meds:

____

____

____

____

Date: ____________

Weight: ____________

Daily Goal: ____________

	Calories	Carbs (g)	Sugars (g)	Fiber (g)	Protien (g)	Fat (g)
Breakfast: Time: ______						
Lunch: Time: ______						
Dinner: Time: ______						
Page Totals:						

Sleep: ______________________

Water: ______________________

Mood: ______________________

	Calories	Carbs (g)	Sugars (g)	Fiber (g)	Protien (g)	Fat (g)
Other Meals / Snacks:						
Page Totals:						

Blood Sugar Log	Before	After	Insulin	Meds
Breakfast				
Lunch				
Dinner				

Activity • Exercise	Duration	Calories	Intensity

Other Notes, Vitamins, Supplements Meds:

____

____

____

____

Date: ________________

Weight: ________________

Daily Goal: ________________

	Calories	Carbs (g)	Sugars (g)	Fiber (g)	Protien (g)	Fat (g)
Breakfast: Time: ________						
Lunch: Time: ________						
Dinner: Time: ________						
Page Totals:						

Sleep: ____________________

Water: ____________________

Mood: ____________________

	Calories	Carbs (g)	Sugars (g)	Fiber (g)	Protien (g)	Fat (g)
Other Meals / Snacks:						
Page Totals:						

Blood Sugar Log	Before	After	Insulin	Meds
Breakfast				
Lunch				
Dinner				

Activity • Exercise	Duration	Calories	Intensity

Other Notes, Vitamins, Supplements Meds:

____

____

____

____

Date: ______________

Weight: ______________

Daily Goal: ______________

	Calories	Carbs (g)	Sugars (g)	Fiber (g)	Protien (g)	Fat (g)
Breakfast: Time: ______						
Lunch: Time: ______						
Dinner: Time: ______						
Page Totals:						

Sleep: ____________________

Water: ____________________

Mood: ____________________

	Calories	Carbs (g)	Sugars (g)	Fiber (g)	Protien (g)	Fat (g)
Other Meals / Snacks:						
Page Totals:						

Blood Sugar Log	Before	After	Insulin	Meds
Breakfast				
Lunch				
Dinner				

Activity • Exercise	Duration	Calories	Intensity

Other Notes, Vitamins, Supplements Meds:

____

____

____

____

Date: ____________

Weight: ____________

Daily Goal: ____________

	Calories	Carbs (g)	Sugars (g)	Fiber (g)	Protien (g)	Fat (g)
Breakfast: Time: ______						
Lunch: Time: ______						
Dinner: Time: ______						
Page Totals:						

Sleep: ______________________

Water: ______________________

Mood: ______________________

	Calories	Carbs (g)	Sugars (g)	Fiber (g)	Protien (g)	Fat (g)
Other Meals / Snacks:						
Page Totals:						

Blood Sugar Log	Before	After	Insulin	Meds
Breakfast				
Lunch				
Dinner				

Activity • Exercise	Duration	Calories	Intensity

Other Notes, Vitamins, Supplements Meds:

____

____

____

____

Date: ____________

Weight: ____________

Daily Goal: ____________

	Calories	Carbs (g)	Sugars (g)	Fiber (g)	Protien (g)	Fat (g)
Breakfast: Time: ______						
Lunch: Time: ______						
Dinner: Time: ______						
Page Totals:						

Sleep: ______________________

Water: ______________________

Mood: ______________________

	Calories	Carbs (g)	Sugars (g)	Fiber (g)	Protien (g)	Fat (g)
Other Meals / Snacks:						
Page Totals:						

Blood Sugar Log	Before	After	Insulin	Meds
Breakfast				
Lunch				
Dinner				

Activity • Exercise	Duration	Calories	Intensity

Other Notes, Vitamins, Supplements Meds:

____

____

____

____

Date: ________________

Weight: ________________

Daily Goal: ________________

	Calories	Carbs (g)	Sugars (g)	Fiber (g)	Protien (g)	Fat (g)
Breakfast: Time: ________						
Lunch: Time: ________						
Dinner: Time: ________						
Page Totals:						

Sleep: ____________________

Water: ____________________

Mood: ____________________

	Calories	Carbs (g)	Sugars (g)	Fiber (g)	Protien (g)	Fat (g)
Other Meals / Snacks:						
Page Totals:						

Blood Sugar Log	Before	After	Insulin	Meds
Breakfast				
Lunch				
Dinner				

Activity • Exercise	Duration	Calories	Intensity

Other Notes, Vitamins, Supplements Meds:

____

____

____

____

Date: ____________

Weight: ____________

Daily Goal: ____________

	Calories	Carbs (g)	Sugars (g)	Fiber (g)	Protien (g)	Fat (g)
Breakfast: Time: ______						
Lunch: Time: ______						
Dinner: Time: ______						
Page Totals:						

Sleep: ____________________

Water: ____________________

Mood: ____________________

	Calories	Carbs (g)	Sugars (g)	Fiber (g)	Protien (g)	Fat (g)
Other Meals / Snacks:						
Page Totals:						

Blood Sugar Log	Before	After	Insulin	Meds
Breakfast				
Lunch				
Dinner				

Activity • Exercise	Duration	Calories	Intensity

Other Notes, Vitamins, Supplements Meds:

____

____

____

____

Date: ________________

Weight: ________________

Daily Goal: ________________

	Calories	Carbs (g)	Sugars (g)	Fiber (g)	Protien (g)	Fat (g)
Breakfast: Time: ________						
Lunch: Time: ________						
Dinner: Time: ________						
Page Totals:						

Sleep: ____________________

Water: ____________________

Mood: ____________________

Other Meals / Snacks:	Calories	Carbs (g)	Sugars (g)	Fiber (g)	Protien (g)	Fat (g)
Page Totals:						

Blood Sugar Log	Before	After	Insulin	Meds
Breakfast				
Lunch				
Dinner				

Activity • Exercise	Duration	Calories	Intensity

Other Notes, Vitamins, Supplements Meds:

____

____

____

____

Date: ______________

Weight: ______________

Daily Goal: ______________

	Calories	Carbs (g)	Sugars (g)	Fiber (g)	Protien (g)	Fat (g)
Breakfast: Time: _______						
Lunch: Time: _______						
Dinner: Time: _______						
Page Totals:						

Sleep: ____________________

Water: ____________________

Mood: ____________________

Other Meals / Snacks:	Calories	Carbs (g)	Sugars (g)	Fiber (g)	Protien (g)	Fat (g)
Page Totals:						

Blood Sugar Log	Before	After	Insulin	Meds
Breakfast				
Lunch				
Dinner				

Activity • Exercise	Duration	Calories	Intensity

Other Notes, Vitamins, Supplements Meds:

____

____

____

____

Date: ____________

Weight: ____________

Daily Goal: ____________

	Calories	Carbs (g)	Sugars (g)	Fiber (g)	Protien (g)	Fat (g)
Breakfast: Time: ______						
Lunch: Time: ______						
Dinner: Time: ______						
Page Totals:						

Sleep: ______________________

Water: ______________________

Mood: ______________________

	Calories	Carbs (g)	Sugars (g)	Fiber (g)	Protien (g)	Fat (g)
Other Meals / Snacks:						
Page Totals:						

Blood Sugar Log	Before	After	Insulin	Meds
Breakfast				
Lunch				
Dinner				

Activity • Exercise	Duration	Calories	Intensity

Other Notes, Vitamins, Supplements Meds:

____

____

____

____

Date: ______________

Weight: ______________

Daily Goal: ______________

	Calories	Carbs (g)	Sugars (g)	Fiber (g)	Protien (g)	Fat (g)
Breakfast: Time: ______						
Lunch: Time: ______						
Dinner: Time: ______						
Page Totals:						

Sleep: ____________________

Water: ____________________

Mood: ____________________

Other Meals / Snacks:	Calories	Carbs (g)	Sugars (g)	Fiber (g)	Protien (g)	Fat (g)
Page Totals:						

Blood Sugar Log	Before	After	Insulin	Meds
Breakfast				
Lunch				
Dinner				

Activity • Exercise	Duration	Calories	Intensity

Other Notes, Vitamins, Supplements Meds:

____

____

____

____

Date: ________________

Weight: ________________

Daily Goal: ________________

	Calories	Carbs (g)	Sugars (g)	Fiber (g)	Protien (g)	Fat (g)
Breakfast: Time: ________						
Lunch: Time: ________						
Dinner: Time: ________						
Page Totals:						

Sleep: ______________________

Water: ______________________

Mood: ______________________

	Calories	Carbs (g)	Sugars (g)	Fiber (g)	Protien (g)	Fat (g)
Other Meals / Snacks:						
Page Totals:						

Blood Sugar Log	Before	After	Insulin	Meds
Breakfast				
Lunch				
Dinner				

Activity • Exercise	Duration	Calories	Intensity

Other Notes, Vitamins, Supplements Meds:

____

____

____

____

Date: ____________________

Weight: ____________________

Daily Goal: ____________________

	Calories	Carbs (g)	Sugars (g)	Fiber (g)	Protien (g)	Fat (g)
Breakfast: Time: ________						
Lunch: Time: ________						
Dinner: Time: ________						
Page Totals:						

Sleep: ____________________

Water: ____________________

Mood: ____________________

	Calories	Carbs (g)	Sugars (g)	Fiber (g)	Protien (g)	Fat (g)
Other Meals / Snacks:						
Page Totals:						

Blood Sugar Log	Before	After	Insulin	Meds
Breakfast				
Lunch				
Dinner				

Activity • Exercise	Duration	Calories	Intensity

Other Notes, Vitamins, Supplements Meds:

____

____

____

____

Date: ____________

Weight: ____________

Daily Goal: ____________

	Calories	Carbs (g)	Sugars (g)	Fiber (g)	Protien (g)	Fat (g)
Breakfast: Time: ______						
Lunch: Time: ______						
Dinner: Time: ______						
Page Totals:						

Sleep: ____________________

Water: ____________________

Mood: ____________________

	Calories	Carbs (g)	Sugars (g)	Fiber (g)	Protien (g)	Fat (g)
Other Meals / Snacks:						
Page Totals:						

Blood Sugar Log	Before	After	Insulin	Meds
Breakfast				
Lunch				
Dinner				

Activity • Exercise	Duration	Calories	Intensity

Other Notes, Vitamins, Supplements Meds:

____

____

____

____

Sugar? Nah, I Am Sweet Enough

Made in the USA
Monee, IL
20 November 2019